Nádia Iara V. dos Santos Ferreira
Glesiane J.Ferreira
Letícia Marotto

Balance and Quality of Life in People with Multiple Sclerosis

Nádia Iara V. dos Santos Ferreira
Glesiane J.Ferreira
Letícia Marotto

Balance and Quality of Life in People with Multiple Sclerosis

A necessary and vitally important analysis for understanding this disease

ScienciaScripts

Imprint

Cover image: www.ingimage.com

This book is a translation from the original published under ISBN 978-613-9-73757-4.

Publisher:
Sciencia Scripts
is a trademark of
Dodo Books Indian Ocean Ltd. and OmniScriptum S.R.L publishing group

120 High Road, East Finchley, London, N2 9ED, United Kingdom
Str. Armeneasca 28/1, office 1, Chisinau MD-2012, Republic of Moldova, Europe
Printed at: see last page
ISBN: 978-620-7-88181-9

Summary

The aim of this study was to analyse the impact of physiotherapy on Balance and Quality of Life (QoL) in people with Multiple Sclerosis (MS). The general aim of this study is to analyse balance and quality of life in MS patients before and after physiotherapeutic intervention. A

The methodology used was initial assessment and reassessment after 12 physiotherapy sessions. The assessment instruments used were the Dynamic Gait Index (DGI), the Berg Balance Scale and the Functional Determination of Quality of Life in MS Scale (DEFU). The results showed

that there was a difference in balance before and after physiotherapy intervention according to the DGI and BERG test scores, with a 5% significance level. With regard to QoL, this study showed that there was no statistically significant difference after 12 physiotherapy sessions.

The conclusion of this study is that physiotherapy is essential in improving the balance of these individuals, but that it is necessary to spend more time with them.

intervention to analyse how physiotherapy affects the QoL of these patients.

Keywords: Multiple sclerosis, Balance, Physiotherapy.

SUMMARY

CHAPTER 1

INTRODUCTION

Considered to be one of the most common pathologies affecting the Central Nervous System, Multiple Sclerosis (MS) is a chronic and progressive disease that mainly affects young adults in their 20s and 40s. It is more prevalent in females, affecting 2 or 3 times more than males, and in the white race (FLORES et al., 2014; AZEVEDO, 2015).

Sir Augustus D'Este first documented reports of Multiple Sclerosis (MS) in 1882, according to Costa et al. (2005). In 1979, Medaer R. recorded the first case of MS, referring to St Lidwina of Schiedam (1380-1433). Lidwina lived in Holland in the 14th century and historical texts reveal that she suffered from a debilitating illness with characteristics compatible with MS (COSTA et al., 2005).

It wasn't until 1868 that the disease was formally identified and described by the eminent French neurologist Jean Martin Charcot. Initially, Charcot called it plaque sclerosis, as he described the hardened, scar-like areas that are found in the Central Nervous System (CNS) of individuals with the disease, as reported by Costa et al. (2005).

It is the most common demyelinating disease of the central nervous system. It is a disease considered to be of autoimmune origin in which activated T cells cross the blood-brain barrier to initiate an inflammatory response, which leads to demyelination and axonal damage (O'SULLIVAN, 2004; NALI et al., 2014). See figure 1 below.

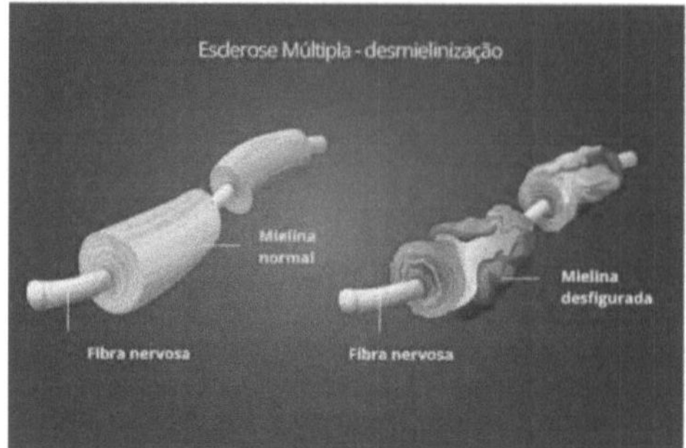

https://images1.minhavida.com.br/imgHandler.ashx?mid=35093

Histological and immunohistochemical studies indicate an extensive area of demyelination of the grey matter in people affected by MS (CALABRESE et al., 2010).

According to Santos in 2010, the initial phase of MS is subtle and is characterised by transient symptoms that last between five days and a week. These characteristics mean that the individual doesn't attach any importance to the first clinical manifestations of the disease, since the symptoms are transitory.

Kumar also described in 2010 that with the progression of MS, the clinical course takes the form of episodes of flare-up and remission of varying duration (from weeks to months or years), characterised by neurological deficits, followed by gradual partial recovery of neurological functions. These relapses tend to diminish as the disease progresses.

Anatomically, MS affects the central nervous system, predominantly the optic nerve, the cervical spinal cord, the brainstem and the periventricular white matter. The lesions are multifocal with different temporal evolution and vary in size, these lesions are seen as a "black hole", the darker the lesions, the greater the tissue damage (CARDOSO, 2010; O SULLIVAN, 2004).

Despite the existence of various terms in the literature used to classify MS, in general the disease is subdivided into different clinical types:

a) **Relapsing-remitting** (RR): onset of the disease characterised by complete recovery or sequelae and residual deficits begin to accumulate due to the repetition of crises.
b) **Primary Progressive** (PP): progression of the disease from the beginning, symptoms develop gradually and there are no outbreaks, improvements occur in less time.
c) **Secondary Progressive** (SP): initially characterised by exacerbations-remissions, followed by progression of impairment and minimal remissions.
d) **Progressive Exacerbation** (PE): progressive disease from the start, but without clear acute exacerbations, which may or may not have some recovery or remission, the latter being less frequent (O'SULLIVAN, 2004; GOODIN et al., 2002; ALVES et al., 2014).

The main mechanisms responsible for initiating the disease are still unknown (MARIN et al., 2014). Thomaz et al. (2005) describe MS as a degenerative disease of the CNS. It is a chronic and progressive disease of unknown aetiology, but it is thought to be the result of a genetic predisposition related to some environmental factor, also with a presumed autoimmune origin and characterised by multifocal inflammation of T lymphocytes, which affects the CNS, mainly the white matter, through demyelinating lesions.

The clinical manifestations depend on the affected areas of the CNS and are the result of conduction block or conduction delay due to demyelination of large segments or axonal damage. The

Lhermitte's is a transient symptom described as an electric shock with dorsal irradiation from active or passive flexion of the neck (OLIVEIRA, 2014).

SYMPTOMS

The main motor symptoms include

Spasticity - a motor disorder characterised by increased muscle tone, dependent on speed, associated with exacerbation of the myotatic reflex (VIVANCOS et al., 2007). It is related to decreased functional capacity, limited joint range of motion, pain, increased metabolic energy expenditure and impaired activities of daily living. Spasticity can also cause stiffness, dislocations, contractures and joint deformities. However, this symptom should not be completely eliminated but rather modulated, as this increased tone can contribute to joint stabilisation, improved posture, easier transfers and decubitus changes (SOMMERFELD, 2004; O'SHEA, 2008).

Muscle spasm - this is a sustained, involuntary and usually painful muscle contraction that cannot be relieved voluntarily. The degree of contraction of the muscle in spasm exceeds its functional needs. It can be caused by any painful condition, or somatic or visceral dysfunctions. Skeletal muscle spasm causes and aggravates existing pain (YENG, 2003).

Contracture - an involuntary, unconscious, painful and permanent contraction that is localised in a muscle or muscle bundle and remains spontaneous with rest (FREITAS et al, 2005).

Gait disorders - are present in 87 per cent of confirmed cases of the disease, causing motor difficulties. Changes in gait can manifest even in patients with minimal degeneration of motor function and without any functional restrictions. Some abnormalities found early on in the gait pattern are: reduced progression speed, shorter strides and prolonged double support phase.

Gait disorders that affect people with MS include:

- **Ataxic gait**: characterised by an increased base of support, reduced stride length and speed, impaired rhythm and excessive foot lifting.
- **Equine gait**: foot drop with toes pointing downwards, causing the toes to scratch the ground and necessitating raising the leg to a higher position than normal when walking.
- **Scissor walk**: legs slightly bent at the hip and knees bent, with the knees and thighs knocking together or crossing in a scissor-like movement.
- **Spastic gait**: stiff gait with foot dragging caused by a long muscle contraction on one side.

Fatigue - is an important symptom in individuals with MS and has repercussions on their activities of daily living, being one of the most frequent and disabling symptoms, affecting around 80-90% of patients (INDURUWA et al., 2012).

Fatigue can be persistent or related to physical activity or minor degrees of mental exertion and is often the initial symptom of an exacerbation (O' SULLIVAN, 2004).

It is defined as a subjective and non-specific symptom, such as a feeling of deep physical or mental tiredness, loss of energy or even exhaustion, with characteristics different from those observed in depression or muscle weakness. It can appear at any time of the day, including at rest, and is present in all forms of the disease, being more severe in the progressive forms. Fatigue is also present in muscle groups that are less affected, such as the dorsal and respiratory muscles (LATIMER- CHEUNG et al., 2013).

It has a significant impact on practically every aspect of an individual and their daily functioning. It is generally measured by self-report. The measurement scales included in this analysis are: Fatigue Severity Scale, Fatigue Impact Scale among others (LATIMER- CHEUNG et al.,2013).

Latimer-Cheung also notes that fatigue can bring a feeling of physical and/or mental exhaustion, lack of vigour or tiredness that can occur at different times of the day, including at rest, and can be present in various muscle groups and although it manifests itself in all forms of MS, its occurrence is more intense in the progressive forms.

According to Comi et al. (2001), fatigue is an overwhelming feeling of tiredness, lack of energy or a sense of exhaustion, often present even at rest. Patients have the feeling that the effort required to perform actions is disproportionately high. As a result, patients tend to reduce their physical activity. Fatigue is usually greatest in the second half of the day and worsens with stress.

Cerebellar and bulbar symptoms such as:

Balance and coordination deficits - imbalance is one of the most common symptoms in MS, causing unsteadiness in walking and favouring falls (NILSAGARD et al., 2015).

There is some evidence that progressive resistance and aerobic training have positive effects on balance in people with MS whose level of disability is mild or moderate (ALMEIDA et al., 2007).

Intentional tremor - This is also called cerebellar tremor, essential tremor or spinocerebellar ataxia. This vagueness of the name is due to the fact that the anatomopathological bases of intentional tremor indicate cerebellar involvement and there is an intentional component. It's a slow tremor, it happens in action and worsens when it hits a target, the intentional tremor is sometimes not rhythmic. During sleep and complete relaxation it disappears (KOLLER, 1984; FINDLEY, 1988). We can also see a rhythmic oscillation of the head and/or trunk called titubation (FAHN, 1972).

Dysphagia - difficulty swallowing is common in people with this disease, especially in those with more severe neurological impairment. Dysphagia has been identified in around 90 per cent of MS patients. The relapsing-remitting form often has mild and moderate dysphagia, while severe dysphagia is often found in the progressive forms (FERNANDES, 2013).

Difficulty breathing - Respiratory complications are described as one of the frequent causes of death in people with MS. Lung impairment occurs due to muscle weakness, including the respiratory muscles.

Although lung involvement is more severely affected in the advanced stages of MS, the respiratory muscles are affected even in the early stages. There are studies proposing that the reduced strength of these muscles plays an important role in the development of fatigue in MS patients. We should therefore be aware of the importance of a well-established Pulmonary Rehabilitation Programme from the beginning of the disease, aimed at optimising respiratory muscle strength and function with expiratory and inspiratory muscle training (TAVEIRA, 2011).

Eye changes - visual disturbances are common in MS and in most cases are the first clinical sign of the disease. Although optic neuritis has been the most frequent finding, we can highlight the possibility of other ocular alterations preceding or accompanying the development of the disease, such as: Decreased visual acuity, Nystagmus, Diplopia **and** Scotomas, popularly known as blurred vision (DE OLIVEIRA, 1998).

Urinary incontinence or retention - we depend on the proper functioning of nerve connections for adequate bladder performance, since the correct transmission of messages to and from the brain is necessary for perfect filling and emptying of the bladder (GOMES, 2010). However, MS causes damage to neurons and hardened plaques are formed in these cells, causing this transmission to be interrupted or to occur slowly (GUIMARÃES, 2017). Patients have symptoms of urinary incontinence and/or retention, as well as enuresis (loss of urine during sleep), difficulty initiating urination, pollakiuria (increased urination) and a feeling that the bladder is not emptying (FRIA, 2013).

Sexual dysfunction - occurs in up to 80 per cent of women and up to 90 per cent of men, and is therefore a prevalent symptom of MS. In both sexes, the most frequent sexual deficit is decreased libido. The most common complaint in women is altered orgasm, while in men it is common to complain of erectile dysfunction (MOTA, 2015).

Sensory Symptoms

As far back as 1872, one of Charcot's patients described complaints of pain and sensory discomfort, but only recently have these complaints been recognised as a frequent and disabling symptom (BEISKE et al., 2004; THOMPSON,2001). According to Frankel, altered sensitivity is common in MS patients, and patients need to be aware of pain, temperature, cracks in the skin and pressure areas due to impaired sensitivity. For patients restricted to bed or a wheelchair, it is important to use cushions and water mattresses to relieve pressure, thus avoiding bedsores (FRANKEL, 2004).

Sensory Reeducation becomes an important point in the treatment of these patients, as it maximises the full sensory potential. Principles of sensory re-education training include: presentation of targeted discriminations by repeating tasks, such as placing objects with different weights and textures in the affected hand and asking for their definition, progression from easy to more difficult discriminations and careful exploration of stimuli with obstructed vision (KALRON et al., 2013).

Sensory symptoms resulting from MS include:

Numbness - is one of the most common signs of a Multiple Sclerosis outbreak. The patient complains of difficulty using their hands, such as writing, holding an object, buttoning a shirt, among other activities of daily living, due to the "numbness" that can affect not only the hands, but also other parts of the body (AME, 2016).

Paresthesia - is a symptom characterised by the sensation of numbness or tingling in some part of the body. Paresthesia can affect the lower and upper limbs and their extremities (feet and hands). Symptoms such as weakness, burning or a sensation of cold or heat may appear. In addition, paresthesia can cause pain that manifests itself as if you were getting pricks. This can lead to a loss of feeling in the affected limb, which can make walking, for example, more difficult (VELOSO, 2017).

Dysaesthesia - The term *"dysestheaia"* originates from the Greek and means **"abnormal sensation".** It consists of the appearance of unpleasant sensations, burning, tingling, itching, or other largely painful discomfort, which are not necessarily caused by any stimulus, but in some situations are distorted perceptions of real stimuli. Some examples are: the sensation of pain when putting on or taking off clothes, brushing your hair and the continuous tingling sensation in your fingers and toes. Dysaesthesias can also occur as a feeling of pressure in the chest, abdomen and around the back. They manifest more frequently after exercise or exertion and as a result of the change in temperature, they tend to worsen when patients try to sleep (FIGUEROBA, 2018).

Musculoskeletal pain - often most observed in the hips, lower limbs and upper limbs, especially when muscles, ligaments and tendons remain inert for some time. Musculoskeletal pain can originate due to muscle weakness, imbalance and spasticity (ABEM 2014).

Emotional symptoms

Depression - it is estimated that a third of people with MS suffer from depression or suicidal thoughts. A study by Nieto-Barco et al. (2008) found a very high rate of depression in MS patients. This is one of the emotional symptoms frequently found in people with this disease.

The origin of depression in MS is probably multifactorial, involving psychosocial and biological factors (ZARZON et al, 2001). The psychological basis of the symptoms of depression in MS is found in the fear and frustration of progressive incapacity and the unpredictability of the course of the disease, while the organic cause is probably related to a disconnection at a cortical or subcortical level in the projection areas of the limbic system (ZARZON et al, 2001).

Depression in individuals with MS is characterised by anger, worry, irritability, pessimism, hopelessness, general loss of energy, sleep disturbances, weight loss, lack of interest, isolation, feelings of guilt and self-deprecation, sexual dysfunction, difficulty concentrating and memory difficulties, the latter three of which may be masked by the MS symptoms themselves (LANA-PEIXOTO et al., 2002; KESSELRING & KLEMENT, 2001).

Cognitive problems - approximately 50% of people with MS suffer from neuropsychological deficits (LANDRO et al., 2004). Memory is the most frequently impaired cognitive function (KESSELRING & KLEMENT, 2001). MS impairs memory both in terms of acquiring new information and retrieving previously processed information; the meta-memory function is impaired, while procedural memory remains intact (FEINSTEIN, 2004).

However, other cognitive areas are affected, such as: image reproduction, spatial-visual processing, reading aloud, motor speed and reaction time, as well as abstract reasoning and verbal fluency (KESSELRING & KLEMENT, 2001; FEINSTEIN, 2004).

Cognitive impairment can have a negative effect on the quality of life of these individuals, since they have less chance of getting a job that is considered relatively stable, they have difficulties in carrying out household chores, they have practically no social life and generally become more dependent on others in Activities of Daily Living (ADLs) when compared to other individuals affected by MS but who do not have cognitive problems (KESSELRING & KLEMENT,

2001).

The results of the changes in cognition caused by the progression of MS can be mitigated through physiotherapy, which aims to provide a better structure and organisation to patients' lives and mitigate the deleterious effects of the disease at a cognitive level (FEINSTEIN, 2004).

CHAPTER 2

EPIDEMIOLOGY/PREVALENCE AND INCIDENCE

The estimated number of people with MS increased from 2.1 million in 2008 to 2.3 million in 2013. This increase can be attributed in part to the increased survival of people with MS and the general population. It may also be due to improvements in diagnosis and the creation of clinical registries, improving communication about this pathology (BROWNE et al.2013).

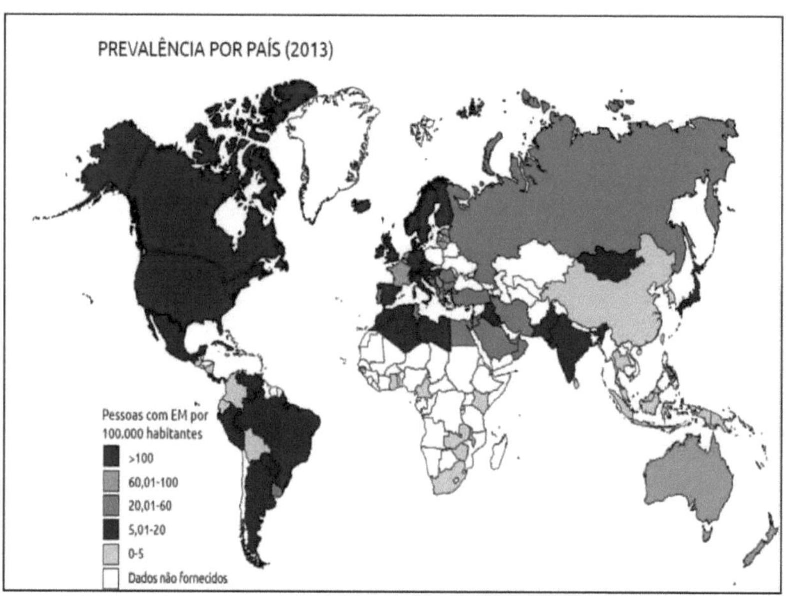

Fig.2: Prevalence of MS by country in 2013.
Source: Browne et al., (2013) © www.atlasofms.org

MS has a wide variation in incidence and prevalence around the world. With less than 5 cases per 100,000 inhabitants, South America is considered to have the lowest prevalence of MS, with a higher incidence in European and North American countries. In Brazil, there is a higher incidence of the disease in the South and Southeast. In the north-east, the prevalence is 10 cases per 100,000 inhabitants. In the south-east this prevalence rises to 12 to 18 per 100,000 inhabitants. In the centre-west region, the prevalence ranges from 4.41 per 100,000 inhabitants to 19 per 100,000 inhabitants and in the south the prevalence is the highest in the country, ranging from 14 to 27 per 100,000 inhabitants (MACHADO et al., 2012).

Approximately 10,376 people in Brazil are undergoing treatment, but data from the Brazilian Multiple Sclerosis Association (ABEM) show that more than 30,000 people are affected. Brazil is considered to have a low prevalence of the disease, but there are regions with a medium prevalence, such as São Paulo, Belo Horizonte and Botucatu. It is speculated that this difference between the various regions of Brazil is partly due to our genetic diversity and our rate of miscegenation (GRZESIUK, 2006). Analyses of population migration show that individuals who migrate from low-risk areas to high-risk areas, especially before the age of 15, have an incidence similar to that of the population of the country that received them, suggesting the presence of a protective factor in the region of origin or a harmful factor in the new region (CORREALE & GAITAN, 2015). It is suggested that in the last 20 years there has been an increase in the incidence of MS, but it is believed that this increase is due to greater recognition and diagnosis of the disease (DEAN, 2007).

CHAPTER 3

ETIOLOGY

The main mechanisms responsible for initiating the disease are still unknown (MARIN et al., 2014). Thomaz et al. (2005) describe this disease as having an unknown aetiology, but it is thought to be the result of a genetic predisposition related to some environmental factor, also with a presumed autoimmune origin.

MS is described as a complex multifactorial disorder, where associated environmental factors interrelate with genetically vulnerable individuals (PUGLIATTI ET AL., 2006). Exposure to Ultra Violet rays or vitamin D deficiency, as well as viral infections, hygiene and smoking are described as possibly responsible for the onset of the disease (ASCHERIO, 2013).

As far as environmental factors are concerned, infectious agents and other microbes play an important role, but we still don't have proof of this association on theoretical grounds (MULTIPLE SCLEROSIS INTERNATIONAL FEDERATION, 2016). With regard to infectious agents, there are two hypotheses: the Poliomyelitis hypothesis and the Prevalence hypothesis. The Poliomyelitis hypothesis defends the existence of a virus that, if the individual is contaminated by it in childhood, acquires a less aggressive and even protective trait of the disease, but if the individual is contaminated by this virus in youth or adulthood, the risk of developing MS is increased (POSKANZER, 1976).

The Prevalence hypothesis is based on studies of the Faroe Islands where the largest epidemic of MS has been recorded, which in turn suggests the existence of a common pathogenic organism in the areas with the highest prevalence (KURTZKE, 1993).

Based on the Poliomyelitis hypothesis, a more general hypothesis was developed and called the Hygiene hypothesis, which defends the idea that exposure to various infectious agents in the first years of life becomes a means of protection against MS, without naming a specific agent (HUNTER, 2000). An environment with a high occurrence of infectious diseases becomes a protective agent against allergic and autoimmune diseases, while a highly hygienic environment increases the incidence of these disorders (BACH, 2002).

Thus, excessive hygiene and the absence of intestinal parasites in childhood may be associated with an increased chance of developing MS. This may explain the high number of allergic and autoimmune diseases in industrialised countries (YAZDANBAKHSH AND MATRICARDI, 2004).

The risk of MS among people who are seronegative for Epstein-Barr Virus (EBV), a virus from the herpes family, is considered to be extremely low. Around 100 per cent of MS patients are seropositive for EBV (BANWELL, 2007; ASCHERIO, 2007). There is a 20 times greater risk of a person who has been infected with EBV in adulthood developing MS than EBV-negative individuals (ASCHERIO, 2007).

Thus, MS is characterised by an autoimmune reaction triggered in susceptible people in response to infection by a multiplicity of organisms, and the older the person infected by these multiple agents, the greater the chances of developing the disease.

With regard to Vitamin D, scholars defend it as an important protective factor for the onset and progression of MS, being an important regulator of immune function and reducing inflammation (CORREALE & GAITAN, 2015). In a review study carried out in 2010 by Solomon and Whitham, which aimed to investigate the interaction between MS and vitamin D, it was observed that severe disability due to outbreaks can jeopardise recommended exposure to the sun's rays, thereby increasing the risk of vitamin D deficiency and consequently worsening symptoms.

With regard to smoking, both the practice of smoking and even exposure to passive smoking have been linked to an increased risk of MS (RHEAD et al., 2016). It has been suggested that active or passive smoking may be a risk factor for changing from a relapsing clinical course to a secondary progressive course. There is an estimated 1.5 for smokers compared to non-smokers (KIMBROUGH, 2012). The means by which tobacco alters the risk and chance of disease progression are not yet known (ABCEM, 2016).

CHAPTER 4

PHYSIOPATHOLOGY

MS is an autoimmune disease whose main mechanism is inflammation of the oligodendrocytes, which in turn are myelin-producing cells (RIVERA; AINGER, 2012). The Myelin Sheath is an electrically insulated layer of nerve fibres in the brain and spinal cord, allowing neurons located close to the axons not to be unduly stimulated (HALL, 2006). This isolation results in the rapid transmission of messages, due to the discontinuous aspect of the myelin sheath making it possible to increase the speed of impulse conduction, as they jump from one node of Ranvier (interruptions in the myelin sheath) to the next, this characteristic is known as the jumping current, giving myelinated axons rapid impulse propagation with a highly reliable transmission factor; the electric current is conducted by the opening of high-voltage Na+ channels found in the nodes of Ranvier, creating a current that spreads from node to node, as shown in the figure below (HALL, 2006).

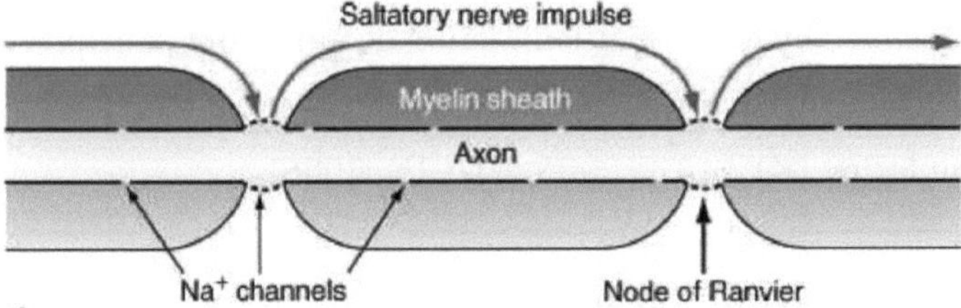

Source: Fauci AS, Kasper DL, Braunwald E, Hauser SL, Longo DL, Jameson JL, Loscalzo J: *Harrison's Principies cf Intemal Medicine* , 17th Edition: http ://www. accessmedicine. com

Fig. 3 - Nerve conduction in myelinated axons

Therefore, if the myelin sheath is damaged, this jumping characteristic is lost, and nerve impulses become slower, as the messages now have to pass along the entire length of the nerve fibres. Therefore, with the destruction of myelin, neurotransmission is impaired, damaging and preventing nerve conduction (ROMÃO et al.,2012).

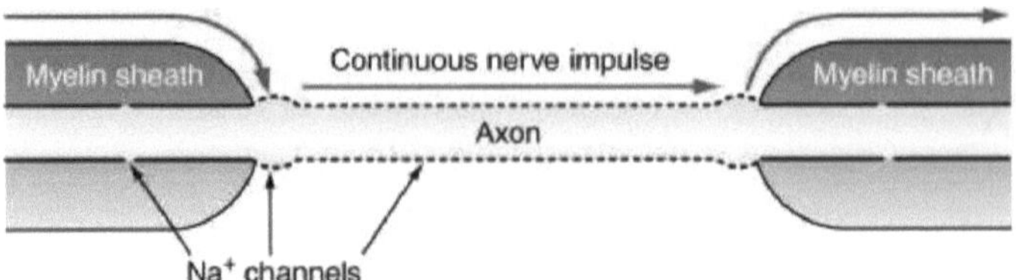

Source. Fauci AS, Kasper DL, Braunwald E. Hauser SL, Longo DL, Jameson JL, Loscalzo J: *Harriscrts Principies Interna! Medicine*, 17th Edition: http://www.accessmedicine.com

Fig. 4 - Nerve conduction in demyelinated axons

The destruction of the myelin sheath can be caused, among other things, by the activation of macrophages and their products. Due to the inflammatory process, macrophages are activated to combat chronic inflammation. This process can make axons demyelinated, leading to inefficient conduction of electrical impulses. When inflammation is reduced, repair mechanisms are activated, which in some cases result in the restoration of damaged myelin, i.e. remyelination. This becomes a cycle (demyelination/remyelination) that can occur several times in the neurons of the Central Nervous System (CNS). When a large region is affected, scars are formed, manifested by the formation of plaques, which can be detected by MRI. If inflammation occurs in the same place repeatedly, the repair mechanism becomes insufficient to promote remyelination, resulting in a permanent lesion (KUMAR, 2005; RUBIN, 2006).

The pathophysiological evolution of MS is therefore inflammatory in nature, resulting in the obliteration of the myelin sheath and occasionally the destruction of axons in the CNS. The area of demyelination forms a typical MS lesion, which is the plaque. It can occur in any region of the CNS and is most commonly found in the white matter, brainstem and spinal cord (SEIXAS et al., 2009).

According to Abreu et al. (2012), the formation of these demyelinating plaques in the CNS is the main pathophysiological feature of Multiple Sclerosis. Several pathological processes are necessary for the formation of these plaques to occur. These processes include disruption of the blood-brain barrier, multifocal inflammation, demyelination, remyelination, loss of oligondendrocytes, reactive gliosis and axon degeneration.

The entire lesional process of MS begins with a cellular immune reaction mediated by the peripheral activation of T lymphocytes that occurs in the blood and lymph nodes, due to some environmental event of unknown origin, perhaps a viral infection or a superantigen. As a result of this activation, the lymphocytes expand, producing different cytokines and increasing the expression of adhesion molecules (ABREU et al., 2012; O SULLIVAN, 2004).

Symptoms result from demyelination and axonal damage, the outcome of which is a decrease in nerve impulse conduction velocity and the interruption of nerve conduction. Symptoms begin to improve due to reduced inflammation and remyelination (MARQUES et al., 2010).

Residual deficits and progressive loss of functionality occur due to limited remyelination capacity and axonopathy (CARDOSO, 2010).

MC DONALDS CRITERIA AND DIAGNOSIS

Since the beginning of the 21st century, the Mc Donald criteria have been important for the early diagnosis of Multiple Sclerosis (MS), with a high degree of specificity and sensitivity. It is important for good patient counselling and early treatment. These criteria were revised in 2005, maintaining the same approach, but simplified, as illustrated in the table below.

CLINICAL PRESENTATION	ADDITIONAL DATA NECESSARY FOR THE DIAGNOSIS OF EM
A) 2 or more outbreaks plus clinical evidence of 2 or more lesions	Only 1 or 2 lesions suggestive of MS on magnetic resonance imaging (MRI)
B) 2 or more outbreaks plus clinical evidence of 1 lesion	Dissemination in space, demonstrated by MRI with Barkhoff criteria, presence of at least 3 of the following 4 characteristics: (a) at least 1 gadolinium-impregnated lesion or at least 9 supratentorial T2 lesions; (b) at least 3 lesions periventricular; (c) at least 1 juxtacortical lesion; (d) at least 1 infratentorial lesion; or MRI with 2 typical lesions and presence of oligoclonal bands on CSF examination; or wait for a new outbreak.
C) 1 outbreak plus clinical evidence of 2 lesions	Spread over time, demonstrated by MRI after 3

	months with new lesions or at least 1 of the old ones impregnated with gadolinium; or wait for a new outbreak.
D) 1 outbreak plus clinical evidence of 1 lesion	Dissemination in space, demonstrated by MRI with Barkhoff criteria or MRI with 2 typical lesions and the presence of oligoclonal bands in the CSF examination. And dissemination over time demonstrated by MRI after 3 months with new lesions or at least 1 of the old ones impregnated with gadolinium or wait for a new outbreak.

Table 1. Mc Donald criteria

Mc Donald's criteria include magnetic resonance imaging (MRI) of the brain, to check for lesions characteristic of demyelination; laboratory tests such as anti-HIV, VDRL and serum vitamin B12, to exclude other pathologies that are similar to MS. If there is any doubt about the diagnosis, a cerebrospinal fluid test is ordered to rule out other diseases, as in the case of suspected Neurolues. If the optic nerve is suspected of being involved in MS, a Visual Evoked Potential test will be required.

(MINISTRY OF HEALTH - Ordinance No. 391 of 5 May 2015).

Expanded Disability Status Scale (EDSS)

The disability of people with MS can be assessed according to a scale developed by John Kurtzke in the mid-1960s, the Expanded Disability Status Scale (EDSS Figure 4). This is a method for quantifying the degree of disability in MS, classifying disability into eight functional systems (FS). As can be seen on the SPEM website (2014), it ranges from 0 (normal neurological examination, no disability) to 10 (confinement to bed, death from MS) and is organised as follows:

- 0.0: Normal neurological examination
- 1.0: No disability, one SF grade 1.5: No disability, two SF grades 1 2.0: Minimum disability in 1 SF (1 SF grade 2, others grade 0 or 1)
- 2.5: Minimum disability in 2 SF (2 SF grade 2, others grade 0 or 1)
- 3.0: Moderate disability in 1 SF (1 SF grade 3, others grade 0 or 1) or slight

disability in 3 or 4 SF (3/4 SF grade 2, others grade 0 or 1). Fully ambulating.

- 3.5: Full ambulation, with moderate disability in 1SF (1 SF grade 3) and 1 or 2 SF grade 2; or 2SF grade 3; or 5 SF grade 2 (others 0 or 1)
- 4.0: Full ambulation, up to 500 m without help or rest (1 SF grade 4, others 0 or 1)
- 4.5: Full ambulation, up to 300 metres without help or rest. With some limitation of activity or requires minimal assistance (1 SF grade 4, others 0 or 1)
- 5.0: Walking up to 200 metres without help or rest. Limitation in daily activities (equivalents are 1 SF grade 5, others 0 or 1; or combination of lower grades exceeding score 4.0)
- 5.5: Walking up to 100 metres without help or rest. Disability preventing full daily activities (equivalents are 1SF grade 5, others 0 or 1; or combinations of lower grades exceeding score 4.0)
- 6.0: Intermittent or constant unilateral assistance with a cane, crutch or support (equivalents are more than 2 SF grades 3+)
- 6.5: Bilateral assistance (equivalents are more than 2 SF grades 3+)
- 7.0: Can't walk 5 metres even with help. Restricted to wheelchair. Transfers from chair to bed (equivalent are combinations with more than 1 SF 4+, or pyramidal grade 5 alone)
- 7.5: Can only take a few steps. Restricted to a wheelchair. Needs help to transfer (equivalents are combinations with more than 1 SF grade 4+)
- 8.0: Restricted to bed, but can stay out of bed. Retains self-care functions; good use of arms (equivalents are combinations of several SF grade 4+)
- 8.5: Constantly confined to bed. Retains some self-care and arm functions (equivalents are combinations of several SF grade 4+)
- 9.0: Patient incapacitated in bed. Can communicate, does not eat, does not swallow (equivalents are mostly FS grade 4+) 9.5: Patient totally incapacitated in bed. Does not communicate, does not eat, does not

swallow (equivalents are almost all SF grade 4+)

- 10.0: Death from multiple sclerosis.

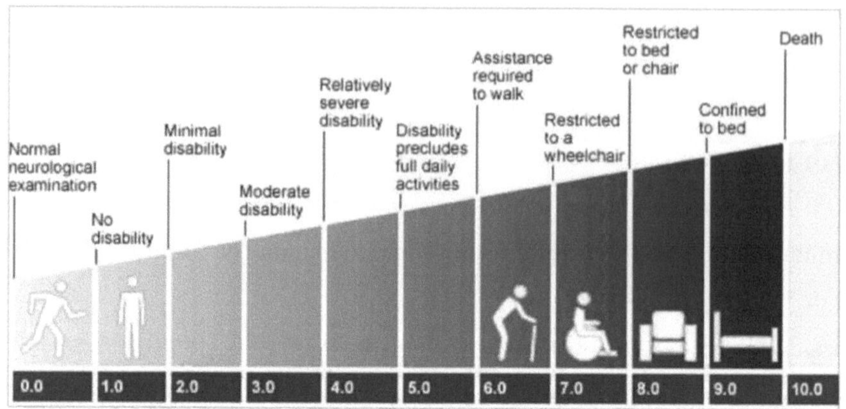

Fig. 4 Expanded Disability Status Scale (EDSS) Source: SPEM 2018

MULTIPLE SCLEROSIS THERAPEUTIC GUIDELINES

In the 1990s, four drugs were tested against placebos, with satisfactory results. There are currently several studies of drugs for the treatment of MS. The first drug used that demonstrated efficacy was Betainterferone, regardless of gender, and it is a reference in the treatment of MS. The use of Betainterferone was tested in patients who had an isolated clinical syndrome with a high risk of developing MS, but without a full diagnosis of the condition. There was a reduction in the rate of relapse, but no benefit in terms of disability or changes in MRI scans.
The use of Glatiramer acetate (40 mg, three times a week) was compared in a randomised clinical trial with the placebo group, in which 1,404 patients took part. The study observed a 34 per cent reduction in relapse and a 34.7 per cent reduction in new lesions on MRI.

In some clinical trials and meta-analyses, Azathioprine has been shown to be effective, even though immunosuppressants are not the first treatment option. Mitoxantrone has been avoided because it has shown a low safety profile in case series.

Long-term use of corticosteroids is not recommended, nor is combining them with other drugs as they do not show any benefit in treatment. According to five meta-analysed studies with 215 patients, there was no difference between the use of oral and intravenous corticosteroids.

In a clinical trial with 1,008 patients followed for three years, there was no efficacy in combining Betainterferone with Glatiramer. Natalizumab is the drug of choice in cases of therapeutic failure of Interferon or Glatiramer (immunomodulators), where the persistence of outbreaks and the progression of the disease are characterised by therapeutic failure. Before Natalizumab can be prescribed, Betainterferone and Glatiramer must have been tried. The condition for using Natalizumab is that the drug must not be combined with any other immunomodulator or immunosuppressant, as there has been a high occurrence of the serious adverse reaction Progressive Multifocal Leukoencephalopathy (PMLE).

Clinical trials and meta-analyses found that there was no advantage in adding statins to betainterferone therapy compared to betainterferone monotherapy.

It was observed in a clinical trial that the addition of cholecalciferol to betainterferon treatment was not significant between the two groups of cholecalciferol or placebo, but a lower number of nerve root lesions was observed (T1).

Fingolimod, a sphingosine 1-phosphate receptor modulator, is used by patients with RRMS who present with disabling outbreaks while taking Betainterferone or Glatiramer and who have a contraindication to the use of Natalizumab.

The therapeutic use of Fingolimod is related to the incidence of delays in atrioventricular conduction, often first-degree atrioventricular blocks, with a prolonged PR interval. Second-degree atrioventricular blocks, usually Mobitz type I (Wenckebach), were noted in less than 0.2 per cent after its marketing. The most frequent adverse reactions with the use of Fingolimod with an incidence of 10% or more at a dose of 0.5 mg were headache, increased liver enzymes, diarrhoea, cough, flu and back pain.

Methylprednisolone is advised to be used when the patient is in an MS flare-up and can be administered for 3-5 days, during which time other drugs should be discontinued.

Betainterferone is superior to other therapeutic options, with absence of flare-ups, absence of clinical progression and absence of progression on magnetic resonance imaging.

Treatment failure or the appearance of intolerable adverse effects determines the length of treatment or drug change. In order to determine treatment failure, two or more outbreaks in a 12-month period of a moderate or severe nature are required, or with an EDSS evolution of 1 point, or the evolution of lesions in disease activities. These criteria are applied to any MS treatment.

The expected benefits of regular use of the drug are symptomatic improvement of the disease, a reduction in the frequency and severity of recurrences and a reduction in the number of hospital admissions.

(MINISTRY OF HEALTH - Ordinance No. 391, of 5 May 2015).

CHAPTER 5

QUALITY OF LIFE

Understanding the cognitive and emotional difficulties of people with MS is an indispensable factor when deciding on a rehabilitation programme, as is understanding their lifestyle, personal preferences, family relationships, work and their role in the community (PEDRO, 2008).

Therefore, in order to arrive at a correct assessment of the state of health of MS patients, this cannot be restricted solely to the parameters of incapacity and disability. Professionals need to understand the strong relationship between health and Quality of Life (CARVALHO, 2003).

Quality of Life is subjective and there is no widely recognised concept or definition. Various factors influence Quality of Life and affect health, including physical, psychological and social conditions (SILVA et al., 2015).

This list of factors, however, is growing. In recent years, in addition to those related to health, fundamental elements of life and how people react are also being related, in other words, how people perceive situations involving friends, family, work and also the unforeseen events of life that happen on a daily basis (SILVA et al., 2015).

The term Quality of Life is broad, encompassing the physical, psychological, socio-cultural, economic and spiritual domains in relation to the state of health and well-being of individuals. The concept is multidimensional, i.e,

addressing various aspects of human life. The term Quality of Life has been expanded and modified over the years and has come to mean social development in terms of education, health and leisure, as well as economic issues (SILVA et al., 2015).

It was in 1920 that the term Quality of Life first appeared, but it was only publicised in 1960, taking into account policies related to interests in the search for a better standard of living, concerning economic factors (SILVA et al., 2015).

The World Health Organisation (WHO) defines QoL as: "an individual's **perception of** their position in life, taking into account their culture and values and in relation to their goals, expectations, standard of **living, and main concerns" (TORRES et aL, 2013).**

It is well known that MS impairs the psychological and functional integrity of various areas including neurological, psychological and social functions, among others, in very young people and those of full working age, causing fear and a sense of insecurity about the future. It is therefore necessary to measure Quality of Life in all aspects of the disease and the repercussions on the daily lives of these patients.

A study carried out by Quitanilha (2012) with 13 patients using the Functional Determination of Quality of Life in Multiple Sclerosis Scale (DEFU) concluded that people affected by this disease have a significant negative impact on their Quality of Life.

Pereira et al (2012) applied the Berg Balance Scale and DEFU to 4 individuals with MS, and found an improvement in balance with the Frankel exercises, but no improvement in quality of life.

This can be explained by the fact that they don't accept the disease because they are young people in the midst of productive activity.

The assessment of QoL in Multiple Sclerosis patients is extremely important because, as we have seen, QoL encompasses social, physical and mental aspects that are related to the individual's perception of their condition, including the treatment of their disease, so QoL measurement scales are being considered increasingly important with regard to the assessment, progression of the disease, treatment and management of care provided to MS patients (BAUNSTARCK et al., 2013).

Studies carried out with Multiple Sclerosis patients have shown that there is a reduction in QoL in all its dimensions. This confirms the concept that in the rehabilitation of these patients, the interaction of a multidisciplinary team is essential to meet all their demands, going beyond drug treatment, i.e. it is important to draw up a treatment programme that assists the individual in their bodily, cognitive, emotional and social functions (ALMEIDA et al., 2007).

McCabe and McKern in 2002 assessed the QoL of 381 people with MS and 291 healthy people. It was shown that people with MS experienced lower levels of QoL compared to healthy people, both for subjective dimensions of all QoL domains and for coping with problems and seeking social support.

As well as improving the psychological side of individuals, physical activity physically conditions those who practise it and this physical conditioning improves physical fitness, which is an important factor in carrying out everyday activities (OLIVEIRA et al., 2014).

The principles for promoting quality of life for people with MS

The 10 principles are:

1. People with MS have full capacity to participate in decision-making in their communities during the monitoring and treatment of the disease.
2. People with MS have access to medical care, treatments and therapies suited to their needs.
3. People with MS have access to a range of age-appropriate care services,

enabling them to work as independently as possible.

4. People with MS have the information and services they need to maintain positive health habits and a healthy lifestyle.
5. People with MS have access to the community through accessible public transport and assistive technology for personal cars.
6. Families and carers receive information and support to ease the impact of MS
7. Support systems and services are available to enable people with MS to remain employed for as long as they are productive and want to work.
8. The rights and services intended for people with special needs are available to those who need them, providing an adequate standard of living and flexibility that allows them to adapt to the mutation of the disease, which is characteristic of MS.
9. MS does not restrict the education of patients, their families or their careers.
10. Accessibility, both of public buildings and the availability of accessible houses and flats, is essential for the autonomy of people with MS (WORLD HEALTH ORGANISATION, 2008).

The term "Quality of Life" has various aspects, ranging from a popular concept, widely used today - in relation to feelings and emotions, personal relationships, professional events, advertising, politics, health strategies, social performance, among others - to the scientific point of view, with various definitions in the medical literature (GILL, 1994).

In terms of its application in medical literature, the term Quality of Life is associated with various definitions, such as health conditions and social functioning. Health-related Quality of Life and Subjective State of Health are concepts related to the subjective evaluation of the patient and the repercussions of the state of health on the possibility of living fully (FLECK et al., 1999).

From this perspective, quality of life reflects people's perception that their needs are being met or that they are being denied the opportunities to achieve happiness and self-fulfilment, regardless of their physical state of health or social and economic conditions (WHO, 1998).

BALANCE

Balance is, according to Cook (2003), the ability to maintain the centre of gravity within the base of support.

Tookuni et al (2005) define balance as "the maintenance of the centre of gravity, which must be within the area of the body's support base and which receives constant adjustments from the musculoskeletal system". Balance requires the interaction of multiple sensory-motor processes (visual, vestibular, proprioception) in order to generate coordinated movements aimed at keeping the centre of mass within the limits of stability (PALTAMAA et al., 2012).

In order to carry out activities of daily living, individuals need to be able to balance, which is an essential factor for human well-being. "Coordination is directly linked to this aspect because it is responsible, among other things, for maintaining posture, which is one of the factors responsible for an individual's balance" (DELIBERATO, 2007).

According to a study carried out in 2008 by Rodrigues et al, "imbalance is the biggest complaint of patients with Multiple Sclerosis, showing vestibular dysfunction in most cases". The main objective of this study was to evaluate the effects of physiotherapy on the Balance and Quality of Life of patients with Multiple Sclerosis and concluded that: "The balance and quality of life of individuals with MS improved significantly with targeted physiotherapy intervention."

A systematic review by Mann et al in 2009, which aimed to investigate the influence of physical exercise programmes on body balance, concluded "that the training that showed the best results was that which used a combination of strengthening, stretching and coordination, with 12 sessions being sufficient for young individuals and 20 sessions for the elderly". It is concluded that this training is the most appropriate, as all the objective studies carried out evaluating this practice have had significant results.

According to a study carried out in 2013 in Bahia, people with MS have reduced balance and a high risk of falls, which leads to reduced functional capacity. In addition, there is a reduction in the performance of their activities of daily living due to the fear of falling (DA FONSECA et al., 2013).
In 2007, Cattaneo carried out a study with 44 MS patients using the Berg Balance Scale, which showed a significant improvement in the balance of these patients.

CHAPTER 6

MULTIPLE SCLEROSIS AND PHYSIOTHERAPY

In order to minimise the limitations and complications imposed by MS and optimise functionality, physiotherapy improves quality of life, as it promotes a significant improvement in balance and movement, as well as maintaining muscle strength (ALVES et al., 2014).

A study carried out by Rodrigues et al (2008), which aimed to assess the improvement of MS patients through physiotherapy, included the participation of 10 patients, who underwent physiotherapy three times a week and followed a physiotherapy protocol drawn up by the author. This study reported an improvement in balance and quality of life in these individuals, demonstrating that the monitoring of MS patients through physiotherapy aimed at specific alterations promotes greater functionality and quality of life". In this way, the authors encourage physiotherapy for individuals with MS and emphasise its importance.

The practice of therapeutic exercises as one of the resources of Physiotherapy promotes an increase in V02 max. , better glycaemic control, increased muscle mass, improved self-esteem and self-confidence, improving patients' quality of life (MORADI et al., 2015).

Gutierrez et al (2005) showed that exercise significantly improves the general condition of people with MS. Participation in a structured resistance training programme has positive effects on gait, balance and level of fatigue, as well as cognition.

A systematic review by Paltamaa et al (2012) showed that progressive resistance exercises and balance training have positive effects on improving the balance of patients with mild or moderate disability.

Muscle weakness and fatigue contribute to a reduction in these patients' daily activities, which results in muscle impairment due to inactivity. Physiotherapeutic interventions aimed at improving muscle strength and endurance in individuals with MS are limited. Therapeutic exercise has been avoided in these patients for many years, due to the increase in body temperature and fatigue that can act as a trigger for a new flare-up (MORADI et al., 2015; INDURUWA 2012; GULICK; GOODMAN 2006).

In a study carried out by Oliveira et al in 2014, the aim of which was to characterise physiotherapeutic procedures and analyse the effectiveness of physiotherapy in these individuals, the author states that for some time MS patients were discouraged from practising physical activity.

This measure was adopted in order to conserve energy, control fatigue and mitigate the risk of new outbreaks, but a sedentary lifestyle has had negative repercussions, such as an increased risk of heart disease and reduced functional capacity (OLIVEIRA et al., 2014).

The practice of physical activity by MS patients has increased significantly in recent years. Several studies have shown that this practice improves balance, functional capacity and consequently the Quality of Life of these patients, as exercise can have positive effects on physical functioning, without any negative effects on the symptoms of Multiple Sclerosis (OLIVEIRA et al., 2014; MOLT et al., 2012).

In a study carried out by Kalron et al in 2015, it was found that a programme of exercises aimed at improving balance and, consequently, gait, brought benefits to MS patients. Physiotherapy, through a well-established programme, has the following main objectives:

- Preventing complications
- Empowering independence
- Maintain mobility
- Maintain proper posture
- Maximising self-determination and Quality of Life.

Physiotherapy helps to improve walking, maintain and prevent fractures and deformities, especially when it comes to impairments secondary to MS. Regular mobility exercises prevent contractures and help maintain limb function. Long-term treatment is aimed at maintaining mobility and preventing the individual from becoming wheelchair dependent at an early stage (WEINER; GOETZ, 2003).

CHAPTER 7

OBJECTIVES

General objective

To analyse Balance and Quality of Life in patients with multiple sclerosis, before and after physiotherapeutic intervention.

Specific objectives

a) To compare balance before and after physiotherapy intervention.

b) To see if there is a relationship between balance deficit and decline in Quality of Life.

MATERIAL AND METHOD

This is an exploratory and quantitative applied case study.

A bibliographical review was carried out using scientific articles selected from the Pubmed, Medline and Scielo databases, published between 2000 and 2015, in English and Portuguese.

Key words: multiple sclerosis; quality of life; physiotherapy; balance.

The study included patients diagnosed with MS, of both sexes, under the age of 65 and attending the Emescam Physiotherapy School Clinic, who agreed to take part in the study by signing an informed consent form (Appendix B). Patients who had visual or hearing problems that affected their balance, wheelchair users or any other problem that might make it impossible for them to actively participate in the study, and patients who missed physiotherapy sessions more than three times were excluded.

This study was approved by the Research Ethics Committee (CEP) of the Escola Superior de Ciências da Santa Casa de Misericórdia de Vitória (EMESCAM) under CAAE registration: 47027215.2.0000.5965. The confidentiality of the information extracted from the medical records was ensured by not identifying the patients by name, who were identified numerically preceded by the letter P (P 01, P 02, etc.). The information was kept under the responsibility of the researcher in charge and will remain in her custody for a period of five years. The data

The data collected was sent to Emescam's Statistics Department for descriptive analysis and presented in percentage form.

The norms established in the Guidelines and Regulatory Norms for Research Involving Human Beings of Resolution 466 were respected. Authorisation for the research site was granted by the signing of a Letter of Consent by the Technical Director responsible for the EMESCAM Physiotherapy School Clinic (Appendix C).

The methodology consisted of an assessment before and after physiotherapy intervention, using the Dynamic Gait Index (DGI) to assess dynamic balance. The DGI was developed by Shumway-Cook et al. in 1997 with the aim of assessing peripheral vestibular alterations, dynamic balance, mobility, activities of daily living and the risk of falling (CASTRO et al., 2006).

The scale consists of dynamic tests that encourage vestibular stimuli in the course of walking with obstacles, steps, etc. It is made up of 8 items with 4 alternatives, ranging from 0 to 3 points, where 0 indicates severe impairment and 3 indicates normal performance of the function, the scale has a maximum score of 24 points, indicating a risk of falling when the index is less than or equal to 19 points (CASTRO et al., 2006).

DGI walking tasks: Gait performed by the individual at normal speed, acceleration and deceleration, cephalic rotation movement, cephalic flexion-extension movement, axial body rotation movement, overcoming an obstacle (shoe box), going around an obstacle, going up and down stairs (CASTRO et al., 2006).

Dynamic Gait Index (DGI)

1- Walking on a flat surface

Instructions: Walk at your normal speed from here to the next marker (6 metres).

Classification: Tick the lowest category that applies

(3) Normal: Walks 6 metres, without aids, at a good speed, no evidence of imbalance, normal gait.

(2) Mild impairment: walks 6 metres, at a slow speed, with minimal deviations, or uses walking aids.

(1) Moderate impairment: Walk 6 metres, slow speed, abnormal gait pattern, evidence of imbalance.

(0) Severe impairment: Cannot walk 6 metres unaided, major gait deviations or imbalance.

2) Gear change

Instructions: Start by walking at your normal pace (1.5 metres), when I say "fast", walk as fast as you can (1.5 metres). When I say "slow", walk as slowly as you can (1.5 metres).

Classification: Tick the lowest category that applies

3)) Normal: Able to change gait speed without loss of balance or deviations. Shows a significant difference in gait between normal, fast and slow speeds.

(2) Mild impairment: Able to change speed but has slight gait deviations, or has no deviations but cannot significantly change gait speed, or uses a walking aid.

(1) Moderate impairment: Only makes small adjustments to walking speed, or is able to change speed with significant deviations in gait, or changes speed and loses balance but is able to recover it and continue walking.

(0) Severe impairment: Cannot change speed, or loses balance and looks for support on the wall, or needs to be supported

3. Gait with horizontal movements (rotation) of the head

Instructions: Start by walking at your normal pace. When I say "look right", turn your head to the right side and keep walking forwards until I say "look left", then turn your head to the left side and keep walking. When I say "look forwards", keep walking and look forwards again.

Classification: Tick the lowest category that applies.

(3) Normal: Performs head turns smoothly, with no change in gait.

(2) Mild impairment: Performs head turns smoothly, with a slight change in gait speed, i.e. with minimal change in gait progression, or uses a walking aid.

(1) Moderate impairment: Performs head turns with a moderate change in walking speed, slows down, or staggers but recovers and is able to continue walking.
(0) Severe impairment: Performs the task with severe gait disturbance, i.e. staggering off the path (about 38cm), loses balance, stops, looks for support on the wall, or needs to be supported.

4. Gait with vertical movements (rotation) of the head

Instructions: Start by walking at your normal pace. When I say "look up", lift your head and look up. Keep walking forwards until I say "look down" then tilt your head down and keep walking. When I say "look forwards", keep walking and look forwards again.

Classification: Tick the lowest category that applies

(3) Normal: Performs head turns without altering gait.

(4) Mild impairment: Performs the task with a slight change in gait speed, i.e. with minimal change in gait progression, or uses a walking aid.

(5) Moderate impairment: Performs the task with a moderate change in walking speed, slows down, or staggers but recovers and is able to continue walking.

(6) Severe impairment: Performs the task with severe gait disturbance, i.e. staggering off the path (around 38cm), loses balance, stops, looks for support on the wall, or needs to be supported.

5. Walking and turning on your own body axis (pivot)

Instructions: Start walking at your normal pace. "When I say 'turn round and stop', turn as quickly as you can in the opposite direction and remain stationary facing (this point) your starting point." **Rating:** Tick the lowest category that applies
(3) Normal: Turns the body safely within 3 seconds and stops quickly without losing balance.
(2) Mild impairment: Turns the body safely for longer than 3 seconds and stops without losing balance.
(1) Moderate commitment: Turns slowly, needs to take several small steps to regain balance after turning the body and stopping, or needs verbal cues.
(0) Severe impairment: Cannot turn body safely, loses balance, needs help to turn and stop.

6. Running over an obstacle

Instructions: Start walking at your normal speed. When you reach the shoebox, run over it, don't round it, and keep going. **Rating: Score** the lowest mark that applies
(3) Normal: Able to pass over the box without altering the speed of travel, there is no evidence of imbalance.
(2) Mild impairment: Able to pass over the box, but needs to slow down and

adjust steps to safely pass the box.
(1) Moderate commitment: Can step over the box, but needs to stop and then step over the obstacle. May need verbal cues.
(0) Severe impairment: Cannot perform the task without help.

7. Walking around obstacles
Instructions: Start walking at your normal speed. When you reach the first cone (about 1.80 metres away), go around it to the right. When you reach the second cone (1.80 metres after the first), go round it to the left.
Classification: tick the lower category that applies

(3) Normal: Able to walk around the cones safely, without changing walking speed; no evidence of imbalance.
(4) Minimal impairment: They are able to walk around both cones, but need to reduce their walking speed and adjust their stride to get past them.
(5) Moderate impairment: Able to pass through the cones, but needs to significantly reduce walking speed to perform the task.
(6) Severe impairment: Unable to pass the cones, trips over them and needs physical help.
8. Steps
Instructions: Climb these steps the way you do at home (i.e. using the handrail if necessary). When you reach the top, turn round and go down again.
Classification: tick the lower category that applies
(3) Normal: Alternating feet, without using the handrail.
(2) Minimal compromise: Alternating feet, but needs to use the handrail.
(1) Moderate impairment: puts both feet on the step, needs to use the handrail.
(0) Severe impairment: Can't do it safely.

Total Score (Maximum = 24)
The Berg Balance Scale was created by Katherine Berg in 1992 and translated and adapted into Portuguese by Miyamoto et al. The aim of the Berg scale is to assess balance, thus determining the risk of falls. It is made up of coordination activities, balance, ability to change position, assessment of patient transfers, among others (MIYAMOTO et al., 2004).

It is based on 14 common items of daily life, where each item has 5 alternatives ranging from 0 to 4 points, with 0 being the inability to perform the requested action and 4 being the total ability to perform the function. The maximum score on the Berg scale is 56 points, where a cut-off value of 45 points is considered a predictor of falls, and an index of 36 points or less is associated with a 100 per cent risk of falls. Therefore, the higher the score, the lower the risk of falls (MIYAMOTO et al., 2004).

This scale assesses the individual's balance in 14 situations, representative of everyday activities, such as: standing up, getting up, walking, leaning forward, transferring, turning around, among others. The maximum score to be achieved is 56 points and each item has an ordinal scale of five alternatives ranging from 0 to 4 points, according to the degree of difficulty (MIYAMOTO et al.,2004).

Berg Balance Scale

1. **Sitting to standing**

INSTRUCTIONS: Please stand. Try not to use your hands as support.
( ) 4 able to stand unaided and stabilise independently
( ) 3 able to stand independently using their hands
( ) 2 able to stand using their hands after several attempts
( ) 1 needing minimal help to stand or stabilise
( ) 0 need for moderate or maximum assistance to stay upright

2. **Standing without support**

INSTRUCTIONS: Please stand for two minutes without holding on to anything.
() 4 able to stand safely for 2 minutes
() 3 able to stand for 2 minutes with supervision
() 2 able to stand for 30 seconds without support
() 1 need several attempts to remain unsupported for 30 seconds
() 0 unable to stand for 30 seconds without assistance
If the subject is able to stand for 2 minutes without support, score maximum points in the sitting without support situation. Go on to item 4.

3. **Sitting without back support but with feet flat on the floor or on a stool**

INSTRUCTIONS: Please sit with your arms crossed for 2 minutes.
() 4 able to sit safely for 2 minutes
() 3 able to sit for 2 minutes under supervision
() 2 able to sit for 30 seconds
() 1 able to sit for 10 seconds
() 0 unable to sit without support for 10 seconds

4. Standing to sitting

INSTRUCTIONS: Please sit down.

( ) 4 sits safely with minimal use of hands
( ) 3 controls descent using hands
( ) 2 rests the back of the legs on the chair to control the descent
( ) 1 sits independently but has uncontrolled descent
( ) 0 needs help to sit up

5. Transfers

INSTRUCTIONS: Ask the subject to move from a chair with an armrest to one without an armrest (or a bed).

( ) 4able to pass safely with minimal use of hands
( ) 3 able to pass safely with the use of bare hands
( ) 2able to pass with verbal cues and/or supervision
( ) 1need assistance from a person
( ) 0 need for two-person assistance or supervision for safety

6. Standing without support with eyes closed

INSTRUCTIONS: Please close your eyes and remain still for 10 seconds.

( ) 4 able to stand safely for 10 seconds
( ) 3 able to stand safely for 10 seconds with supervision
( ) 2 able to stand for 3 seconds
( ) 1 unable to keep eyes closed for 3 seconds but remain standing
( ) 0 need for help to avoid falling

7. Standing without support with feet together

INSTRUCTIONS: Please keep your feet together and stand without holding on

( ) 4 able to stand with feet together independently safely for 1 minute
( ) 3 able to stand with feet together independently safely for 1 minute with supervision
( ) 2 able to stand with feet together independently and hold for 30 seconds
( ) 1 needing help to maintain position but able to stand for 15 seconds with feet together
( ) 0 need of help to hold the position but unable to hold it for 15 seconds

8. Reach forwards with your arms outstretched while remaining upright

INSTRUCTIONS: Keep your arms extended at 90 degrees. Extend your fingers and try to reach as far as possible. (The examiner places a ruler at the end of your fingers when your arms are at 90 degrees. The fingers should not touch the ruler while performing the task. The measurement recorded is the distance the fingers can reach while the subject is leaning forwards as far as possible. If possible, ask

the subject to perform the task with both arms to avoid trunk rotation).
( ) 4 able to reliably reach over 25cm (10 inches)
( ) 3 able to reach above 12.5cm (5 inches)
( ) 2 able to reach over 5cm (2 inches)
( ) 1 able to achieve but needs supervision
( ) 0 loss of balance during attempts / need for external support

9. Pick up an object from the floor from a standing position
INSTRUCTIONS: Pick up a shoe/slipper located in front of your feet ( ) 4 able to pick up the slipper easily and safely
( ) 3 able to pick up the slipper but needs supervision
( ) 2 unable to pick up the slipper but can reach 2-5cm (1-2 inches) from the slipper and maintain balance independently
( ) 1 unable to catch and needs supervision while trying
( ) 0 unable to try / needs assistance to prevent loss of balance or fall

10. Standing, turn and look back over your right and left shoulders
INSTRUCTIONS: Turn and look back over your left shoulder. Repeat for the right. The examiner can take an object to look at and place it behind the subject to encourage them to turn.
( ) 4 looks back from both sides with adequate weight shift
( ) 3 looks back for both on one side only, the other side shows less weight shift
( ) 2 only turns both ways but maintains balance
( ) 1 needs supervision when turning
( ) 0 needs assistance to prevent loss of balance or falling

11. Turn 360 degrees
INSTRUCTIONS: Turn completely round in a full circle. Pause. Do the same in the other direction
( ) 4 capable of turning 360 degrees safely in 4 seconds or less
( ) 3 able to safely turn 360 degrees to one side in 4 seconds or less
( ) 2 able to turn 360 degrees safely but slowly
( ) 1 needs supervision or verbal guidance
( ) 0 needs assistance while turning

12. Alternate feet on a step or stool while standing without support
INSTRUCTIONS: Place each foot alternately on the step/bench. Continue until each foot has touched the step/bench four times.
( ) 4 able to stand independently and safely and complete 8 steps in 20 seconds
( ) 3 able to stand independently and complete 8 steps in more than 20 seconds
( ) 2 able to complete 4 steps unaided but with supervision
(   ) 1 able to complete more than 2 steps requiring minimal effort

assistance
( ) 0 needs assistance to prevent falling / unable to try

13. Stand without support with other foot in front
INSTRUCTIONS: (SHOW TO SUBJECT - Place one foot directly in front of the other. If you realise that you can't put your foot directly in front of it, try taking a step wide enough so that the heel of your foot remains in front of the toe of your other foot. (To get 3 points, the length of the step can exceed the length of the other foot and the width of the base of support can approach the subject's normal stepping position).
(   ) 4 able to position the foot independently and maintain it for 30 seconds
( ) 3 able to position the foot in front of the other independently and hold for 30 seconds
( ) 2 able to take a small step independently and hold it for 30 seconds
(   ) 1 needs help to take the step but can keep it for 15 seconds
( ) 0 loss of balance while stepping or standing

14. Stand on one leg
INSTRUCTIONS: Stand on one leg as long as you can without leaning on it
( ) 4 able to lift the leg independently and hold for more than 10 seconds
( ) 3 able to lift the leg independently and maintain between 5 and 10 seconds
(   ) 2 able to lift the leg independently and hold for 3 seconds or more
(   ) 1 tries to lift his leg and is unable to maintain it for 3 seconds, but stands independently
( ) 0 unable to try or needs assistance to avoid falling

(   ) TOTAL SCORE (maximum = 56)

The Functional Determination of Quality of Life in MS Scale (DEFU) was used to measure quality of life. The Functional Assessment of Multiple Sclerosis (FAMS) was developed by Cella et al. in 1996 as a specific scale to quantify the state of health of MS patients (MENDES et al., 2004).

This scale was translated and adapted into Portuguese in 1996 as the Scale for Functional Determination of Quality of Life in Patients with Multiple Sclerosis (DEFU). They used a generic questionnaire developed for cancer patients as a basis, adding questions about symptoms and problems related to MS. The original English version consists of 59 items, 44 of which are used to obtain the score. The remaining 15 items are presented because they provide relevant clinical and social information, but should not be used to obtain the final score (MENDES et al., 2004).

In its final form, the DEFU is made up of 6 sub-items valid for analysis: mobility (7 items), symptoms (7 items), emotional state (7 items), personal satisfaction (7 items), thinking and fatigue (9 items) and social and family situation (7 items). The format of the answers allows scores of 0 to 4 for each item, in a Likert-type format, with the reverse score being considered for questions constructed in a negative way. In this way, higher scores reflect a better quality of life. The five 7-item subscales allow for scores ranging from 0 to 28 and the 9-item subscale (thinking and fatigue) has scores ranging from 0 to 36 (MENDES et al., 2004).

To validate it, the DEFU scale was translated into Portuguese by two bilingual people, one of whom spoke English as their mother tongue. The scale was then translated into English and a consensus was reached. The final format of the scale was maintained, with 6 sub-items and 44 valid questions to obtain the score (MENDES et al., 2004).

DEFU

SCALE OF FUNCTIONAL DETERMINATION OF QUALITY OF LIFE IN MULTIPLE SCLEROSIS

	Iten"	Never	A little	Sometimes	Many Times	Always
Mobility	1. i have problems due to my condition listai, in manlef my 1,imitia '	0	1	2	3	**4**
	2 I can work from home	0	1	2	3	**4**
	3. wood for walking*	0	1	2	3	4
	4. imltacfles in my social voa'	0	1	2	3	4
	5. My legs are strong	0	1	2	3	**4**
	6. I'm embarrassed in public places'	0	1	2	3	4
	1. I made plans because of my illness '	0	1	2	3	4
Symptoms	8. I feel nauseous'	0	1	2	3	**4**
	9. I'm in pain'	0	1	2	3	**4**
	10. I feel ill'	0	1	2	3	**4**
	11. I feel weak'	0	1	2	3	**4**
	12. I have joint pain'	0	1	2	3	**4**
	13. I've got dtxee on my head'	0	1	2	3	4
	14. muscle pain'	0	1	2	3	4
Emotional stat	15. I'm sad '	0	1	2	3	**4**
	16. I'm losing faith in the fight against my illness'	0	1	2	3	4
	17. I'm capable of living life	0	1	2	3	**4**
	18. I feel like a prisoner of my illness '	0	1	2	3	**4**

e	19 I'm depressed because of my situation'	0	1	2	3	4
	20. I feel useless	0	1	2	3	4
	21. I'm overcome by illness'	0	1	2	3	4
Personal Satisfaction	22.0 I find my work satisfying even at home	0	1	2	3	4
	23. I accepted my illness	0	1	2	3	4
	24. I enjoy what I do when I have fun	0	1	2	3	4
	25. I'm satisfied with my quality of life	0	1	2	3	4
	26. I'm frustrated because of my condition '	0	1	2	3	4
	27. I feel a purpose in life	0	1	2	3	4
	28. I feel motivated to carry out cnlsas	0	1	2	3	4
Thinking And Fatigue	29. I have a loss of energy '	0	1	2	3	4
	30. I feel tired '	0	1	2	3	4
	31. I find it difficult to complete tasks because I'm tired'	0	1	2	3	4
	32. I find it difficult to finish tasks because I'm tired '	0	1	2	3	4
	33. I need a rest during the day'	0	1	2	3	4
	34. I have trouble remembering things'	0	1	2	3	4
	35. I find it hard to concentrate '	0	1	2	3	4
	36. My reasoning is 'ento'	0	1	2	3	4
	37. I find it difficult to learn new tasks'	0	1	2	3	4
Social Situation and Bankruptcy	38. I feel distant from my friends'	0	1	2	3	4
	39. I have emotional support from my family	0	1	2	3	4
	40. support from friends and neighbours	0	1	2	3	4
	41. My family has accepted my illness	0	1	2	3	4
	42. Family communication about the disease is poor '	0	1	2	3	4
	43. My family has trouble recognising my relapse'	0	1	2	3	4
	44. I feel excluded from the facts *	0	1	2	3	4
Annex	45. The side effects bother me * #	0	1	2	3	4
	46. I'm forced to spend time in bed * #	0	1	2	3	4
	47. I feel close to my mate #	0	1	2	3	4
	48. I've had sexual contact in the last year N&o...SIm...	0	1	2	3	4
	If I'm satisfied with my sex life #	0	1	2	3	4
	49. The medical team is accessible to my questions #	0	1	2	3	4
	50. I'm proud of how I'm coping with the disease *	0	1	2	3	4
	51. I feel nervous* #	0	1	2	3	4
	52. I'm worried that my illness will get worse* #	0	1	2	3	4
	53. I'm sleeping well * #	0	1	2	3	4

After the first assessment, physiotherapy intervention began, which consisted of balance exercises with a Swiss ball, trampoline, imbalance board, gait training, circuits, strengthening lower limb muscle groups, stretching, Frenkel exercises and Proprioceptive Neuromuscular Facilitation.

The research was carried out at the Multiple Sclerosis Extension Project, which operates at the Physiotherapy School Clinic of the School of Sciences of the Santa Casa de Misericórdia de Vitória, ES (Emescam), from 12/11/2015 to 11/02/2016, with a frequency of one session per week, each session lasting approximately 40 minutes, totalling 12 sessions. At the end of the last session, the patients were reassessed and the scales and test were applied again.

PHYSIOTHERAPEUTIC INTERVENTION

Examples of exercises performed to train balance, proprioception and muscle strength:

- *p* Alternate positioning of the feet to a specific target, using markings on the floor;
- Stand up and sit down on a specific count;
- Rotate under a specific count;
- Weight transfer;
- Walking sideways and forwards (parallel lines were used to control foot positioning, stride length and stride width).

Exercises were also carried out to improve proprioception using the Swiss ball, elasticated bed and unbalance board. To gain ROM, the patients performed stretching exercises. To improve muscle strength, Proprioceptive Neuromuscular Facilitation (PNF) exercises were carried out, which have the ability to teach and carry out a therapeutic programme with richer and more elaborate exercises, not only stimulating the muscles, but the whole body as a whole. Frenkel exercises were used to improve balance and gait, a series of activities with progressive and rhythmic difficulty, aimed at improving proprioceptive control and consequently functional movement.

The research was carried out at the Multiple Sclerosis Extension Project at the Emescam Physiotherapy School Clinic in Vitória, Espírito Santo, from 12/11/2015 to 11/02/2016, once a week, with each session lasting approximately 40 minutes, totalling 12 sessions. After this period, the patients were reassessed and the scales and test were applied again.

Results

Balance before and after physiotherapy treatment was compared using descriptive statistics and the non-parametric Wilcoxon test for paired samples. The result of the Wilcoxon test indicated that there was a difference in balance according to the DGI and BERG test scores, with a 5% significance level.

Table 2. Balance comparison

	Minimum	Maximum	Average	Median	Standard deviation	p-value
CHILDREN	0	6	2	2	2	-
OUTBREAK	1	10	4	4	3	-
DGI before	4,0	24,0	15,5	17,0	5,7	0,042*
DGI then	10,0	24,0	17,8	19,5	5,3	
BERG before	18,0	53,0	43,8	46,5	10,5	0,027*
BERG then	21,0	55,0	42,7	46,0	12,1	

* p-value < 0.05

Applying the DEFU, we found that 80% of the participants in this study had a relatively good quality of life index, while only 20% had lower scores, which indicates a poor QoL index. After 12 physiotherapy sessions, the participants were reassessed and, according to the results of the DEFU, their quality of life did not show any statistically significant difference, as can be seen in Table 1.

Table 3 Comparison of Quality of Life before and after Physiotherapy Intervention

	Average	**Median**	**Standard deviation**
DEFUantes	**74,3**	**76,5**	**11,4**
DEFU_apÓs	**72,3**	**72,5**	**10,6**

DISCUSSION

According to Oliveira et al (2014), the practice of physical activity by MS patients has increased significantly in recent years. Several studies have shown that this practice improves the balance and functional capacity of these patients, as exercise can have positive effects on physical functioning, without any negative effects on the symptoms of Multiple Sclerosis, which was demonstrated in this study where a significant improvement in the patients' balance was obtained, $p<0.05$, both when assessed by the Berg scale when testing static balance and by the DGI when testing dynamic balance.

Studies by Rodrigues et al, (2008) have also shown that imbalance is the biggest complaint of patients with Multiple Sclerosis, concluding in their study that the balance and quality of life of individuals with MS improved significantly with targeted physiotherapeutic intervention. Likewise, the systematic review by Mann et al. in 2009 and the study by Almeida et al. in 2007 showed that conventional physiotherapy combined with balance training is indispensable in physiotherapy protocols for MS patients. A systematic analysis carried out by Paltamaa et al in 2012 showed that progressive resistance exercises and balance training have positive effects on improving the balance of patients with mild or moderate disability. With the aim of assessing and correlating functional disability, fatigue and depression with the QoL of people with MS, Ribeiro et al (2014) carried out a study and concluded that QoL in individuals with MS is influenced by several factors, including age, fatigue and depression. However, functional disability caused by the disease was not found to have a significant influence on QoL, corroborating this study. Studies on QoL in patients with MS are an important tool for assessing the impact of the disease on the daily lives of these patients, given that the evolution of MS involves individual factors and not just criteria of incapacity and disability (MIYAMOTO, 2004). As well as health-related factors, QoL also relates to fundamental elements of life and how people react, i.e. how people perceive situations involving friends, family, work and the unforeseen events of everyday life (TOOKUNI, 2005). In addition to physical factors, other aspects must be considered during physiotherapy intervention so that the treatment plan can meet the real needs of these patients (GULIK, 2006). Of the participants in this study, 80% had higher scores on the Scale of Functional Determination of Quality of Life in MS, which represents a better quality of life, contrasting with the studies by Rodrigues et al (2008) who observed a negative impact on the QoL of the participants in his research, using the same scale. This can be explained by the subjectivity and relativity of QoL, which is defined by the World Health Organisation (WHO) as an individual's personal conception, based on their socio-cultural context, values, dreams, goals, standards and apprehensions to characterise their position in life (TOOKUNI, 2005;

RODRIGUES, 2008). According to a study by Pereira et al. in 2012, no improvement in QoL was observed after 15 physiotherapy sessions, which corroborates the present study where no statistically significant improvement in QoL was observed after 12 physiotherapy sessions. An interesting fact observed in this study was that the relationship between balance and quality of life was inversely proportional when looking at the cases individually, where it was observed that the patient with very good balance, still outside the falls risk zone, showed the worst quality of life index and the patient with the worst balance, already at 100% risk of falls, were the patients who showed the best quality of life, confirming that the negative impact caused by MS can be the result of several factors, and the disability caused by the disease would be just one of them. The fact that you have a chronic, evolving neurological disease with an unpredictable course, gradually incapacitating and so far without a cure, can have a huge impact on patients' lives, even in the early stages (MANN, 2009). The participants in our study did not have a poor QoL when compared to other studies published on the same subject. However, as we set out to see if and how physiotherapy affects the QoL of these individuals, we did not observe any differences before and after the physiotherapy intervention, which may be explained by the age factor, This may be explained by the age factor, as the participants in our study had an average age of 46.2 years, we must take into account that the disease started in the middle of the socio-economic development phase and even in the face of the difficulties peculiar to a chronic disease and so far without a cure, they had an optimistic attitude towards these difficulties. As shown in the results presented, physiotherapy improves the balance and functionality of people affected by multiple sclerosis, but it was not possible to observe statistically significant changes in quality of life in this study, which can be explained by the multidimensional and subjective concept that encompasses quality of life. Balance is only one aspect of these individuals' lives.

The limitations of this study were the short time interval between the first and second assessments, with only 12 physiotherapy sessions, few participants in the study and the presence of outbreaks during the study, which prevented people from attending physiotherapy sessions.

Further studies should be carried out with a longer physiotherapy intervention period and a larger number of patients in order to better observe the real impact of physiotherapy on the quality of life of individuals with MS and the possible impact of physiotherapy on this social situation.

CHAPTER 8

CONCLUSION

This study shows that physiotherapy is essential for improving balance and functional independence in MS patients, as quantified by the scores on the Berg balance scale and the Dynamic Gait Index (DGI).

It was not possible to observe significant changes in quality of life in this study, which can be explained by the multidimensional and subjective concept that quality of life encompasses. More studies with a longer intervention time and a larger number of participants are needed to measure quality of life and the impact of physiotherapy on patients with multiple sclerosis in order to better assess the impact of MS, using generic and specific instruments together to determine the impact of symptoms in more detail, and to check the impact of drug and non-drug interventions on the QoL perceived by patients. As the disease is not very prevalent, multicentre studies with a larger number of patients could produce more consistent results.

REFERENTIAL

ABCEM. Available at: http://www.abcesclerosemultipla.com.br/ Accessed on: 06/11/18

ALMEIDA S. R. M, Bersuaski K, Cacho E.W.A, Oberg T.D. Eficiência do treino de equilíbrio na Esclerose Múltipla. **Fisioterapia em movimento, Curitiba**. 20(2): 41-48, 2007.

ALVES, B. et al. Multiple Sclerosis: Review of the main treatments for the disease. Saúde e Meio ambiente Revista interdisciplinar, v. 3, n. 2, p. 19-34, jul./dez.2014.

AME Multiple Friends for Sclerosis. **Numbness and tingling**. Available at: https://amigosmultiplos.org.br/esclerose-multipla/sintomas/dormencia-e-tingling

ARNOLD R, Ranchor AV, Sanderman R, Kempen GI, Ormel J, Suurmeijer TP. The relative contribution of domains of quality of life to overall quality of life for different chronic diseases. **Qual Life Res.** 2004;13(5):883-96.

ASCHERIO A, Munger KL. Environmental risk factors for multiple sclerosis, part I: the role of infection. **Ann Neurol** 2007; 61: 288-99.

ASCHERIO, Alberto. Environmental factors in multiple sclerosis. **Expert review of neurotherapeutics,** v. 13, n.sup2, p. 3-9, 2013.

AZEVEDO, Maria Teresa Quitério. **Evaluation of the impact of fatigue on activities of daily living in individuals with multiple sclerosis.** 2015. Doctoral thesis.

BACH, Jean-François. The effect of infections on susceptibility to autoimmune and allergic diseases. New England Journal of medicine, v. 347, n. 12, p. 911920, 2002.

BANWELL B, Krupp L, Kennedy J, et al. Clinical features and viral serologies in children with multiple sclerosis: a multinational observational study. **Lancet Neurol** 2007; 6: 773-81.

BAUMSTARCK, K. et al. Measuring the Quality of Life in Patients with Multiple Sclerosis in Clinical Practice: A Necessary Challenge (Online) France. **Multiple Sclerosis International**, v.2013, n.1, p. 1- 8, 2013.

BRAZIL. Ministry of Health. Clinical Protocol and Therapeutic Guidelines for Multiple Sclerosis - Ordinance No. 391. Brasília, DF: **Ministry of Health,** 5 May 2015.

BEISKE, A. G. et al. Pain and sensory complaints in multiple sclerosis. European Journal of Neurology, v. 11, n. 7, p. 479-482, 2004.

BORGES, Juliana Coelho. **Physiotherapeutic Treatment of the Quadriceps Musculature in Vasto Lateral Distension of a Football Player**. 2002. 58f. Monograph (Degree in Physiotherapy) - Faculty of Biological and Health Sciences, Tuiuti University of Paraná. Paraná.

BROWNE P. et al .Atlas of Multiple Sclerosis 2013: A growing global problem with widespread inequity. **Neurology**. 83(11):1022-1024, September 2014.

CALABRESE, M.; Filippi M.; Gallo, P. Cortical lesions in multiple sclerosis. **Nat. Rev. Neurol**, v. 6, n. 8, p. 438-444, jul.2010.

CARDOSO, FAG. Physiotherapy in multiple sclerosis: relapsing remitting form. **Ver. Movimenta** [online]. 2010[access 15 November 2018]. Available at: www.nee.ueg.br

CARVALHO, Adriana et al. Determination of autoantibodies to myelin antigens in the serum of HLA-DQB1* 0602 patients with multiple sclerosis. Arquivo Neuropsiquiatria, v. 61, n. 4, p. 968-973, 2003.

CASTRO. S. M, Perracini M.R, Ganança F.F. Brazilian version of the Dynamic Gait Index. **Rev Bras Otorrinolaringol.** 72(6):817-825, 2006.

CATTANEO, D. et al. Effects of balance exercises on people with multiple sclerosis: a pilot study. **Clin Rehabil**, v. 21, n. 9, p. 771-781, 2007.

COMI, G. et al. Physiopathology and treatment of fatigue in multiple sclerosis. **Journal Neurol Milan**, v. 248, n. 3, p. 174-179, sep.2001.

CORREALE J,Gaitán MI. Multiple sclerosis and environmental factors . **Acta Neurol Scand** 2015 : 132 (Suppl. 199): 46-55. © 2015 John Wiley & Sons A / S. Published by John Wiley & Sons Ltd.

COOK, A. S.; WOOLLACOTT, M. H. Motor Control: Theory and Practical Applications. 2ª edition. **Barueri** - SP: Manole, p 154, 2003.

COSTA, R. et al The illness of people with multiple sclerosis: perceptions and experiences from the narrative of two clinical cases. **Revista Brasileira em Promoção da Saúde**, vol. 18, núm. 3, 2005, pp. 117-124 Universidade de Fortaleza Fortaleza-Ceará, Brazil.

DA FONSECA, Erika Pedreira et al. Relationship between balance deficit, incidence of falls and functional capacity in patients with multiple sclerosis. **Cadernos de Pós-Graduação em Distúrbios do Desenvolvimento,** v. 13, n. 1, p 47-54, 2013.

DEAN, M Wingerchuk, et al. **The spectrum of neuromyelitis optica**; Lancet Neurol 2007; 6: 805-15.

DE FREITAS, Igor Brum et al. Analysis of muscle injury rates in football athletes from the Clube Internacional de Santa Maria/Novo Horizonte-RS sport club. **Disciplinarum Scientia Saúde**, v. 6, n. 1, p. 81-89, 2016.

DELIBERATO, P. C. P. Exercícios Terapêuticos: Guia Teórico Para Estudantes e Profissionais. 1ª ed. Barueri - SP: **Manole,** 2007.

DE OLIVEIRA, Enedina Maria Lobato; DE SOUZA, Nilton Amorim. Multiple sclerosis. **Neurosciences**, p. 114, 1988.

FAHN S. Differential diagnosis of tremors. **Med Clin North Am** 1972;56:1363- 1375.

FEINSTEIN, Anthony. The neuropsychiatry of multiple sclerosis. **The Canadian Journal of Psychiatry**, v. 49, n. 3, p. 157-163, 2004.

FERNANDES, Alessandro Murano Ferré ert al. Oropharyngeal dysphagia in

patients with multiple sclerosis: do the disease classification scales reflect the severity of dysphagia? Braz. J. otorhinolaryngol. (online). 2013, v. 79, n. 4, p. 460-465.
ISSN 1808-8694. http://dx.doi.org/10.5935/1808-8694.20130082

FIGUEROBA, Alex. Dysaesthesia: what this symptom is, causes and types. Available at: psicologiaymente.com/clínica/disestesia

FINDLEY, LJ. Tremors. Differential diagnosis and pharmacology. In: Jankovic J, Tolosa E (eds). **Parkinson's disease and Movement Disorders**. Baltimore, Urban and Schwarzenberg,1988. p.243-261.

FLECK MPA, Leal OF, Louzada S, Xavier M, Chachamovich E, Vieira G, et al. Development of the Portuguese language version of the

WHO quality of life (WHOQOL-100). **Rev Bras Psiquiatr**. 1999;21(1):19-28.

FLORES FM, Sousa LS, Menezes KM, Copetti F, Trevisan CM. Quality of life in multiple sclerosis patients participating in therapeutic horseback riding. **ConScientiae Saúde** (online) 2014 accessed 12 November 2018; 13(1): 39-46. Available at: http//www.redalyc.org

FRANKEL, D. Multiple Sclerosis. In: UMPHRED, D. A. Reabilitação neurológica. 4th ed. São Paulo: **Manole,** p. 627-647, 2004.

FREITAS, Igor Brum. et al. Analysis of muscle injury rates in football players from the esporte clube internacional de santa maria / novo horizonte - RS. **Disciplinarum Scientia**, Santa Maria, v. 6, p 81-89. 2005.

FRIA, Ana Márcia Pinheiro et al. Urinary dysfunction in a patient with multiple sclerosis. **Rev. Neurocienc**, v. 21, n. 2, p. 247-250, 2013.

GILL TM, Feisntein AR. A critical appraisal of the quality of quality-of-life measurements. **JAMA.** 1994;272(8):619-26.

GOODIN, D. S. et al. Disease modifying therapies in multiple sclerosis. **Neurology**, v. 58, n. 2, p. 169-178, 2002.

GOMES, Cristiano Mendes; HISANO, Marcelo. Anatomy and physiology of urination. **AN Júnior, MZ Filho, & RB dos Reis (Eds.), Fundamental Urology,** p. 29-36, 2010.

GRZESIUK K. Clinical and epidemiological characteristics of 20 patients with multiple sclerosis in Cuiabá - Mato Grosso, Brazil. **Arq. Neuro- Psiquiatr.** 64(3), São Paulo September, 2006.

GUIMARÃES, Jaqueline Pereira; Schoffen, João Paulo Ferreira. Multiple sclerosis: the profile of a mysterious neurological dysfunction. **Revista Uningá Review**, v. 1, n. 1, 2017.

GULIK E.E, Goodman S. Physical activity among people with multiple sclerosis. **International Journal of MS Cares.** 8(4):121-129, 2006.

GUTIERREZ, Gregory M. et al. Resistance training improves gait kinematics in persons with multiple sclerosis. **Archives of physical medicine and rehabilitation.** 86(9):1824-1829, 2005.

HALL, J E. Guyton Physiology Review. 11. **ed. Philadelphia**: Elsevier; 2006.

INDURUWA I, Constantinescu CS, Gran B. Fatigue in multiple sclerosis: a brief review. **J Neurol** Sci.323(1-2): 9-15, 2012.

KALRON, A. et al. Effects of a new sensory re-education training tool on hand sensibility and manual dexterity in people with multiple sclerosis. **Neuro Rehabil**, v. 32, n.4, p. 943-948, 2013.

KESSELRING, Jurg; KLEMENT, Ulrike. Cognitive and affective disturbances in multiple sclerosis. **Journal of neurology,** v. 248, n. 3, p. 180-183, 2001.

KIMBROUGH, Dorlan J. et al. Treatment of neuromyelitis optica: review and recommendations. **Multiple sclerosis and related disorders**, v.1, n. 4, p. 180-187, 2012.

KINGWELL E et al. Incidence and prevalence of multiple sclerosis in Europe: a systematic review. BMC neurology (online). 2013, (accessed 09 November 2018); 13(1):128 Available at: http://bmcneuro.biomedcentral.com

KOLLER WC. Diagnosis and treatment of tremors. Neurol Clin 1984; 2:499-514.

KUMAR V, Abbas A, Fausto N. Robbins & Cotran. **Pathological bases of diseases**. 7. ed. Rio de Janeiro: Saunders; 2005.

KURTZKE JF. Epidemiological evidence for multiple sclerosis as na infection. **Clin Microbiol Rev** 1993;6:382-427.

LANA-PEIXOTO, Marco Aurelio et al. Expanded BCTRIMS consensus for the treatment of multiple sclerosis: III. Evidence-based guidelines and recommendations. **Arquivos de neuro-psiquiatria**, v. 60, n. 3B, p. 881-886, 2003.

LANDRO, Nils Inge; CELIUS, Elisabeth Gulowsen; SLETVOLD, Helge. Depressive symptoms account for deficient information processing speed but not for impaired working memory in early phase multiple sclerosis. **Journal of the neurological sciences**, v. 217, n. 2, p.211-216, 2004.

LATIMER-CHEUNG et al. "Effects of Exercise Training on Fitness, Mobility,Fatigue, and Health-Related Quality of Life Among Adults With Multiple Sclerosis: A Systematic Review to Inform Guideline Development". **Archives of Physical Medicine and Rehabilitation**, v. 94, n.9, p.1800-1828, 2013.

MARÍN, N. et al. Anti-myelin antibodies play an important role in the susceptibility to develop proteolipid protein-in- duced experimental autoimmune encephalomyelitis. **Clinical & Experimental Immunology**, v. 175, n. 2, p. 202-207, Feb.2014.

MCCABE, M. P.; MCKERN, S. Quality of life and multiple sclerosis: comparison between people with multiple sclerosis and people from the general population. **Journal of Clinical Psychology in Medical Settings**, v. 9, n. 4, p. 287-295, 2002.

MANN L, Kleipaul J.F, Mota C.B, Santos S.G. Body balance and physical exercise: a systematic review. **Motriz rev. educ. fís.** 15(3): 713-722, Rio Claro. 2009.

MENDES, M. F. et al. "Validação de escala de determinação funcional da qualidade de vida na esclerose múltipla para a língua portuguesa. **Arq Neuropsiquiatr**, v. 62, n. 1, p. 108-113, 2004.

MIYAMOTO S.T., Lombardi Junior I., Berg K.O., Ramos L.R., Natour J.. Brazilian version of the Berg balance scale. **Braz J Med Biol Res** [Internet]. 2004 [access 2018 November 12]; 37(9): 1411-1421. Available at: www.scielo.br/scielo. doi.org/10.1590/S0100-879X2004000900017

MOTL, R. W. et al. Combined training improves walking mobility in persons with significant disability from multiple sclerosis: a pilot study. **Journal of Neurologic Physical Therapy**, v. 36, n. 1, p. 32-37, Mar.2012.

MORADI, Mahbubeh et al. Effects of Eight-week Resistance Training Programme in Men With Multiple Sclerosis. **Asian journal of sports medicine.** 6(2):1-7, 2015

MOTA, Ana Marta Barreto. **Sexual dysfunction in multiple sclerosis**. 2015. Master's dissertation.

NALI, LHS, et al. Natalizumab treatment for multiple sclerosis: updates and considerations for safer treatment in JCV positive patients. **Arq. Neuro-Psiquiatr.** [Internet]. 2014 Dec [access 2018 November 12] ; 72(12): 960-965. Available at: www.scielo.br/scielo doi.org/10.1590/0004- 282X20140142

NEVES, Marcos Antonio Orsini et al. Physiotherapeutic approach to minimising the effects of taxia in individuals with multiple sclerosis. www.revistaneurociencias.com.br, p. 160, 2007.

NIETO BARCO A, Sánchez López MeP, Barroso Ribal J, Olivares Pérez T, Hernández Pérez MA. [Cognitive impairment in the early phase of multiple sclerosis and its relationship with mood, demographic and clinical variables]. **Psicothema**. Nov 2008; 20(4): 583-8.

NILSAGÂRD, Y. et al. Falls in people with MS-an individual data meta-analysis from studies from Australia, Sweden, United Kingdom and the United States. **Multiple Sclerosis Journal**, v. 21, n. 1, p. 92-100, Jan.2015.

NORTVEDT, M., & Riise, T. (2003). Nortvedt, M., & Riise, T. (2003). The use of quality of life measures in multiple sclerosis resaerch. Multiple Sclerosis, 9, 63-72.

WORLD HEALTH ORGANISATION. **Health promotion: glossary**. Geneva: WHO; 1998.

O'SHEA, T. Michael. Diagnosis, treatment, and prevention of cerebral palsy in near-term/term infants. **Clinicai obstetrics and gynecology**, v. 51, n. 4, p. 816, 2008.

O'SULLIVAN, S. B. Multiple Sclerosis. In: O'SULLIVAN, S. B. Physiotherapy: Assessment and Treatment. 4th ed. Barueri: **Manole**, 2004 844-876.

OLIVEIRA A.C.F.R, Andrade V.S, Gontijo D.T, Barroso S.M. Characterisation and complaints related to occupational performance: considerations of individuals with multiple sclerosis. **Ver. Ter. Ocup**

OLIVEIRA N.G, Bofi T.C, Barbatto L.M, Carvalho A.C. "Analysis of a physiotherapy programme in a group of patients with multiple sclerosis." **MTP&RehabJournal**. 12(1):831-845, 2014.

PALTAMAA J, Sjogren T, Peurala S.H, Heinonen A. Effects of physiotherapy interventions on balance IN multiple sclerosis: A systematic review and META-analysis of randomised controlled trials. **J Rehabil Med.** 44(10):811-823, 2012.

PEDRO LMR, Pais-Ribeiro JL. Psychometric characteristics of instruments that assess quality of life in multiple sclerosis. **Fisioter Pesqui** 2008; 15 (3): 309-314.

PEDRO, L., & Pais-Ribeiro,J. (2006). Review of quality of life instruments in multiple sclerosis. In: I.Leal, J. Pais-Ribeiro & S.Neves, (Edts.). **Proceedings of the 6th National Congress of Health Psychology** (pp.121-126). Lisbon: ISPA

PEREIRA EF, Teixeira CA, Santos A. Quality of life: approaches, concepts and evaluation. **Rev bras Educ Fís Esporte** 2012;26(2):241-50.

POSKANZER DC, Walker AM, Yonkondy J, Sheridan JL. Studies in the epidemiology of multiple sclerosis in the Orkney and Shetland Islands. **Neurology** 1976;26:14 -17

PUGLIATTI, Maura et al. The epidemiology of multiple sclerosis in Europe. **European journal of Neurology**, v. 13, n. 7, p. 700-722, 2006.

QUINTANILHA, R. S.; LIMA, L. R. Evaluation of quality of life in patients with Multiple Sclerosis. **Revista de Enfermagem UFPE**, Recife, v. 4, n. 1, p. 153- 161, 2010.

RIBEIRO BB, Pereira LS, Mello NF, Filippin NT. Relation of functional disability, fatigue and depression with the quality of life of people with Multiple Sclerosis. **Biomotriz** ISSN 2014; 8 (1): 50-64.

RIVERA, F. J.; AIGNER, L. Adult mesenchymal stem cell therapy for myelin repair in multiple sclerosis. **Biological research**, v. 45, n. 3, p. 257-268, 2012.

RHEAD, Brooke et al. Mendelian randomisation shows a causal effect of low vitamin D on multiple sclerosis risk. **Neurology Genetics**, v., n. 5, p. 97, 2016.

RODRIGUES IF, Nielson MBP, Marinho AR. Evaluation of physiotherapy on balance and quality of life in participants with multiple sclerosis. **Rev Neurocienc.** 2008 16(4): 269-274.

ROMÃO, G. P. et al. Assistance to patients with multiple sclerosis: Identified health needs and promotion of a better quality of life. Rev. **Enfermagem Revista**, v. 15, n. 1, p. 72-87, Jan./Apr.2012.

RUBIN E, Gorstein F, Rubin R, Schwarting R, Strayer D. Rubin **Pathology. Clinical and pathological bases of medicine.** 4. ed. Rio de Janeiro: Guanabara Koogan; 2006.

SANTOS FLS, Corrêa NMH, Leal RMP, Monteiro CFS. The experience of the spouse/partner of a person with multiple sclerosis. **Rev.enferm.UERJ** 2010 18(2):229-234.

SEIXAS D, Galhardo V, Sá MJ, Guimarães J, Lima D. Pain in multiple sclerosis: characterisation of a Portuguese population of 85 patients. **Acta médica Portuguesa** (online). 2009 (accessed 12 November 2018); 22(3): 233240. Available at: http//www.actamedicaportugues.com

SILVA, A. S.; FILIPPIN, N. T.; QUATRIN, L. B. Effects of physiotherapy interventions on the balance and functional capacity of individuals with

multiple sclerosis: a literature review. **Disciplinarum Scientia**. Series: Health Sciences, Santa Maria, v. 16, n. 1, p. 35-42, 2015.

SOLOMON, Andrew J: WHITHAM, Ruth H. Multiple sclerosis and vitamin D: a review and recommendations. **Current neurology and neuroscience reports**, v. 10, n. 5, p. 389-396, 2010.

SOMMERFELD, Disa K et al. Spasticity after stroke: its occurrence and association with motor impairments and activity limitations. **Stroke**, v.35,n.1, p. 134-139, 2004.

TAVEIRA, Fernanda Machado; TEIXEIRA, Antonio Lúcio; DOMINGUES, Renan Barros. Respiratory complications in multiple sclerosis. **Rev Bras Neurol**, v. 47, n. 4, p. 16-24, 2011.

THOMPSON, A. J. Symptomatic management and rehabilitation in multiple sclerosis. Journal of Neurology, Neurosurgery & Psychiatry, v. 71, n. 2, p. 2227, 2001.

TOOKUNI, Karla Sayuri; et al. Comparative Analysis of Postural Control in Individuals With and Without Anterior Cruciate Ligament Injury of the Knee. **Acta Ortopedia Brasileira**. 13(3)115-119, 2005.

TOMAZ, A. et al. Signs and symptoms associated with otoneurological alterations diagnosed by computerised vestibular examination in patients with multiple sclerosis. Arq. Neuropsiquiatric, v. 63, n. 3, p. 837-742, 2005

VELOSO, Heloísa Helena Pinho et al. Prevalence of paresthesia resulting from endodontic treatment in the municipality of João Pessoa-PB. **Odontological Journal of Central Brazil,** v. 26, n.79, 2017.

VIVANCOS-MATELLANO F, Pascual-Pascual SI, Nardi-Vilardaga J, Miquel-Rodriguez F, de Miguel-Leon I, Martinez-Garre MC, et al. [Guide to the comprehensive treatment of spasticity]. **Rev Neurol**. 2007;45(6):365-75. Spanish.

WEINER, W. J; GOETZ, C, G. Neurology for the Non-specialist: Basic Fundamentals of **Contemporary** Neurology. 4. ed. São Paulo: Santos, 2003.

WILLIS MK, Robertson NP. Alemtuzumab for the treatment of multiple sclerosis. Ther **Clin Risk Manag** (online). 2015 (accessed 28 November 2018);11:525-534. Available at: www.ncbi.nlm.nih.gov.

WORLD HEALTH ORGANISATION et al. Multiple sclerosis international federation. **Atlas: multiple sclerosis resources in the world**, 2008.

YAZDANBAKHSH, Maria; MATRICARDI, Paolo M. Parasites and the hygiene hypothesis. Clinical reviews allergy & immunology, v. 26, n. 1, p. 15-23, 2004.

YENG, L.T.; KAZIYAMA, H.H.; TEIXEIRA, M.J. Myofascial pain syndrome. **JBA**, Curitiba, v.3, n.9, p.27-43, jan./mar. 2003.

ZARZON, M. et al. (2001). Depression and anxiety in multiple sclerosis. A clinical and MRI study in 95 subjects. **J Neurol**, 248:416-421.

ZEQIRAJ, K., KRUJA, J., KABASHI, S., & MUÇAJ, S. Epidemiological Characteristics and Functional Disability of Multiple sclerosis Patients in Kosovo. **Medical Archives**. 68(3) 178-181, 2014.

MIX
Papier aus verantwortungsvollen Quellen
Paper from responsible sources
FSC® C105338

Printed by Books on Demand GmbH, Norderstedt / Germany